Nurses' Aids Series

MULTIPLE CHOICE

Book 1

NAS
NURSES' AIDS SERIES

Nurses' Aids Series

Multiple Choice Questions
Book 1

Anatomy and Physiology	SHEILA M. JACKSON SRN, SCM, BTA, RNT
Medical Nursing	CHRISTINE M. CHAPMAN BSc(Soc), MPhil, SRN, SCM, RNT
Paediatric Nursing	BARBARA F. WELLER SRN, RSCN, RNT
Surgical Nursing	ELIZABETH J. FISH SRN, ONC, RCNT, RNT
Advisory Editor	CHRISTINE WARD MA

BAILLIÈRE TINDALL · LONDON

A BAILLIÈRE TINDALL book published by
Cassell Ltd.
35 Red Lion Square, London WC1R 4SG
and at Sydney, Auckland, Toronto, Johannesburg
an affiliate of
Macmillan Publishing Co. Inc.
New York

First published 1977
Reprinted 1978, 1979

ISBN 0 7020 0647 5

Printed in Great Britain by
The Whitefriars Press Ltd, London and Tonbridge

Contents

Preface

Objective questions are being increasingly used by examining bodies, sometimes as the only method of examining, more often as one part of a two- or three-part examination. The most commonly used type of objective question is multiple choice, but this book also contains matching-block and assertion/reason questions.

The growing popularity of objective questions is attributable to a number of factors. Because each question is short and quickly answered, it is possible to cover a much greater proportion of the syllabus than can normally be done with the more traditional types of question, and, as the questions are all compulsory, each candidate is answering questions on the same parts of the syllabus and to the same standard as all other candidates. Because the questions do not require written answers, each candidate's performance is unaffected by his or her skill in writing and self-expression and, therefore, reflects more closely his or her knowledge of the subject matter. The multiple choice question, in particular, has been revised and developed over the years to indicate not only students' factual information but their judgement and problem-solving ability as well. Finally, and perhaps most important, a reason for the increased use of the objective-question test is the elimination of subjective judgement and possible 'examiner bias' from the marking.

With the introduction by the General Nursing Council for England and Wales in the autumn of 1977 of objective tests as a part of the written Examination and Assessment, this new addition to the Nurses' Aids Series is meant to provide practice and experience for those preparing for their examinations. The questions in this book are not drawn from any existing bank; they are original and based only upon information contained within the various selected books in the Nurses' Aids Series, and are intended to be used in conjunction with those books.

In *Book 1,* the questions are prepared by the author or, in two instances, by the co-author of the original work. In order to determine the suitability of the questions, they have been scrupulously pretested and revised accordingly to achieve the best possible practice for student and pupil nurses.

Anatomy and Physiology, prepared by Sheila M. Jackson, includes questions that are based on the new approach to learning the subject, with emphasis on the basic scientific principles for a clearer understanding of the chemistry of the body as well as its mechanics. Some of the topics covered are: systems and parts of the body; the blood; the respiratory system; nutrition; the digestive system; the ear; the eye; the reproductive systems.

Medical Nursing, by Christine M. Chapman, is a standard textbook for use during training and for reference afterwards. Her questions are based on the basic principles of nursing care therein and on the latest developments in diagnosis and treatment.

Paediatric Nursing questions are prepared by Barbara F. Weller. They cover the text on the development of the healthy child and the treatment and care of sick children in hospital, including among other areas, infant feeding, the sick neonate and mental and physical handicap.

Surgical Nursing, by Elizabeth J. Fish, is a concise account of the principles and practice of nursing the surgical patient. Miss Fish has drawn her questions from various chapters, giving particular attention to those on admission, preoperative and postoperative care and complications arising after surgery.

Because certain subjects would overlap, for example, from Anatomy and Physiology to, say, Paediatric Nursing, the authors have consulted each other throughout the writing of their sections to avoid as much as possible any repetition. As a result, the questions and chapters are selective rather than comprehensive. The questions are arranged according to the chapter of the book to which they refer, so the reader may use particular chapters for revision before turning to the relevant questions. Conversely, in view of the subject matter involved, the questions can also be used quite independently of the particular books on which they are based.

May 1977

Acknowledgements

The Publisher and Authors wish to extend their grateful appreciation to all those who gave their assistance willingly and enthusiastically to this book. In particular: to Mrs J. Exton-Smith, Director of Nurse Education, Barnet Area School of Nursing; Miss S. Green, Senior Tutor, Queen Elizabeth School of Nursing; Mrs B. E. Hume, Assistant Area Director of Nurse Education, Sefton Area School of Nursing; Mr G. Fremantle, Senior Tutor, North Hertfordshire School of Nursing; and to the many student and pupil nurses who assisted in pretesting; to Miss Vera H. Darling, Examinations and Assessments Officer, General Nursing Council for England and Wales, for sharing her expertise in the history and background of multiple choice questions; and to Miss Nancy Philcox for the preparation of manuscript and matrices.

Instructions for Multiple Choice Questions

An objective question is one in which the possible answers are written out, and the candidate has only to select the correct one; since the answer is predetermined, the questions can be marked by reference to an answer key and no subjective judgement is involved. The most commonly used type of objective question is the multiple choice question; to give you a broader approach to objective questions, you will also find in this book matching-block and assertion/reason questions.

How To Use This Book

Do not look at the questions until you think that you have learned as much as you can of the relevant subject matter. If you are using the questions chapter by chapter, work through the relevant chapter of the book in the Nurses' Aids Series and then attempt the objective questions on that chapter. If you are attempting all the questions in one set at once, do not do so until you have revised the subject matter; then work through all the questions allowing yourself up to $1\frac{1}{2}$ to 2 hours – you will probably not need as long as that. Mark your answer to each question in the book or on a separate piece of paper. When you have answered all questions as well as you can, check your answers by referring to the answer key at the end of the book. Then re-read the parts of the textbook which refer to the questions which you answered incorrectly.

Most of the questions in this book are of the *multiple choice* type. In each of these questions there is a question or incomplete statement followed by FOUR possible answers, only ONE of which is correct. Decide which one is correct and mark it by ringing the letter beside it, e.g.

(a)
(b)
ⓒ
(d)

If you change you mind you can cross out the ring and mark your new choice, e.g.

(a)
ⓑ
ⓧ
(d)

In *assertion/reason* questions the 'stem' consists of an ASSERTION, which may or may not be true, followed by a REASON which may or may not be true and, if true, may or may not be a correct explanation of the assertion. You must decide which of the possibilities is correct, selecting from the following list:

(a) both assertion and reason are true statements and the reason is a correct explanation of the assertion
(b) both assertion and reason are true statements but the reason is not a correct explanation of the assertion
(c) the assertion is true, but the reason is a false statement
(d) the assertion is false, but the reason is a true statement
(e) both assertion and reason are false statements

Mark your choice by ringing the appropriate letter in the same way as for multiple choice.

Each *matching-block* question consists of an introductory statement followed by two lists and a 'match panel' which is to be used to match the items in List 2 to those in List 1, e.g.

A	B	C	D
4	5	3	1

There will be one item in List 2 which is not used.

How Well Did You Score?

The sets of questions in this book have been 'pretested', that is, they have been tried out on samples of up to 200 student or pupil nurses studying the relevant subject matter. If you attempt all the questions in one set at once you can compare your performance with theirs by referring to the following table

	No. of questions	*Average score*	*75% of the students scored more than*	*25% of the students scored more than*
Anatomy and Physiology	100	56	46	64
Medical Nursing	80	47	40	52
Paediatric Nursing	80	44	37	50
Surgical Nursing	90	41	32	49

Anatomy and Physiology

Chapter 6

1. Normal bone growth requires adequate amounts of

    (a) vitamin B
    (b) vitamin D
    (c) iron
    (d) potassium

2. Which of the following is *not* a function of the periosteum?

    (a) to give attachment to tendons
    (b) to supply nourishment to the bone
    (c) to increase bone circumference
    (d) to increase bone length

Chapter 7

3. How many lumbar vertebrae are there?

    (a) 12
    (b) 7
    (c) 5
    (d) 4

Chapter 8

4. The neck of the femur lies

   (a) just above the knee joint
   (b) between the head of the femur and the greater trochanter
   (c) between the greater and lesser trochanters
   (d) between the trochanters and the shaft

Chapter 9

5. The hip joint is an example of

   (a) a pivot joint
   (b) a ball and socket joint
   (c) a double hinge joint
   (d) a gliding joint

Chapter 12

6. The reaction of the blood is

   (a) strongly alkaline
   (b) slightly alkaline
   (c) neutral
   (d) slightly acid

7. The average circulating blood volume in an adult is

   (a) 3–4 litres
   (b) 5–6 litres
   (c) 7–8 litres
   (d) 9–10 litres

8. Oedema can be caused by

    (a) excessive salt intake
    (b) excessive fluid intake
    (c) a deficiency of potassium
    (d) a deficiency of plasma proteins

9. Serum consists of

    (a) blood without red cells
    (b) blood without thrombocytes (platelets)
    (c) plasma without fibrinogen
    (d) plasma without globulin

10. The anti-anaemic factor is composed of

    (a) the intrinsic factor and vitamin B12
    (b) the extrinsic factor and vitamin B12
    (c) the intrinsic factor and folic acid
    (d) the extrinsic factor and folic acid

11. A constituent of human blood which is a rich source of antibodies is

    (a) thromboplastin
    (b) gamma-globulin
    (c) leucocytes
    (d) thrombocytes (platelets)

12. Approximately how many erythrocytes (red cells) are there in one cubic millimetre of blood?

    (a) 5000
    (b) 50 000
    (c) 500 000
    (d) 5000 000

13. Which of the following substances is normally present in the blood?

    (a) thrombokinase
    (b) thrombin
    (c) fibrin
    (d) prothrombin

14. Which of the following is *not* a function of the blood?

    (a) to provide materials for the manufacture of glandular secretions
    (b) to regulate body temperature
    (c) to cushion the brain and spinal cord
    (d) to arrest haemorrhage through clotting

15. A patient has blood belonging to group AB. He should be able to receive blood from

    (a) group AB only
    (b) any other blood group
    (c) groups A, B and AB only
    (d) groups AB and O only

16. Which of the following is *not* a polymorphonuclear leucocyte?

    (a) granulocyte
    (b) neutrophil
    (c) basophil
    (d) monocyte

17. Thrombocytes (platelets) are important in

    (a) fighting infection
    (b) maintaining normal haemoglobin levels
    (c) the blood clotting mechanism
    (d) erythrocyte (red cell) formation

Chapter 13

18. The apex beat of the heart can be most accurately located

    (a) above the xiphisternum
    (b) below the left nipple
    (c) in the fifth left intercostal space
    (d) in the seventh left intercostal space

19. The interior of the heart is lined with

    (a) pericardium
    (b) endocardium
    (c) myometrium
    (d) endomysium

20. The blood vessels which communicate with the left atrium of the heart are called

    (a) the pulmonary arteries
    (b) the coronary veins
    (c) the venae cavae
    (d) the pulmonary veins

21. The sinu-atrial node (pacemaker of the heart) is situated in the

    (a) wall of the right atrium
    (b) atrioventricular bundle (bundle of His)
    (c) atrioventricular node
    (d) wall of the right ventricle

22. The function of valves in blood vessels is to

    (a) prevent the blood flowing in the wrong direction
    (b) push the blood on
    (c) prevent blood entering areas where it is not required
    (d) reduce the rate of flow when the body is at rest

23. The sounds of the heart are caused by

    (a) blood flowing through narrow orifices
    (b) the ventricles contracting
    (c) the valves opening
    (d) the valves closing

24. Three of the following vessels carry deoxygenated blood. Which does *not*?

    (a) pulmonary artery
    (b) pulmonary vein
    (c) coronary sinus
    (d) portal vein

25. The pulse is

    (a) a wave of blood travelling along the veins
    (b) a wave of distension travelling along the arteries
    (c) the recoil of the arteries following distension
    (d) compression of an artery against a bone

Chapter 14

26. Blood is carried to the liver by

    (a) the hepatic artery and the mesenteric artery
    (b) the mesenteric artery and the portal vein
    (c) the hepatic vein and the hepatic artery
    (d) the hepatic artery and the portal vein

27. Oxygenated blood is carried to the lungs by the

    (a) brachial arteries
    (b) bronchial arteries
    (c) intercostal arteries
    (d) aorta

28. The blood circulates through the veins because of

    (a) suction as the heart contracts
    (b) suction as expiration occurs
    (c) pressure due to muscular contraction
    (d) pressure from blood in the arteries

29. When taking the blood pressure using a stethoscope diastolic blood pressure is recorded

    (a) when the first sound is heard
    (b) when the sound becomes muffled
    (c) when the sound disappears
    (d) when the second sound is heard

30. Which of the following are *all* essential in the maintenance of arterial blood pressure?

    (a) the viscosity of the blood, the total blood volume, the ventricular output
    (b) the viscosity of the blood, the elasticity of the arterial walls, the lymphatic drainage
    (c) peripheral resistance, suction due to inspiration, total blood volume
    (d) peripheral resistance, massage by muscular contraction, total blood volume

Chapter 15

31. The function of the lymphatic capillaries is to carry

    (a) food and oxygen from the blood stream to the cells
    (b) waste products from the cells to the blood stream
    (c) tissue fluid from the interstitial spaces to the lymphatic vessels
    (d) intracellular fluid from the cells to the blood stream

32. One function of lymphatic nodes is to

    (a) filter the blood of waste products
    (b) filter the blood of bacteria
    (c) filter the lymph of waste products
    (d) filter the lymph of bacteria

33. Which of the following is *not* a function of the spleen?

    (a) the manufacture of red blood cells
    (b) the manufacture of white blood cells
    (c) the breakdown of red blood cells
    (d) the manufacture of antibodies

Chapter 16

34. The cavity of the nose is lined with ciliated epithelium.
    The function of the cilia is to

    (a) moisten the air
    (b) entrap some of the dust
    (c) move the mucus into the pharynx
    (d) warm the air

35. The maxillary sinuses lie

    (a) within the ethmoid bone
    (b) below the orbit
    (c) in the midline of the frontal bone
    (d) in the body of the sphenoid bone

36. Tidal volume is the amount of air breathed in and out
    during normal quiet respiration. This is about

    (a) 500 ml
    (b) 1000 ml
    (c) 1500 ml
    (d) 2000 ml

37. *Assertion*   *Reason*
    The right main bronchus   the heart lies a little
    is wider, shorter and   *because*   to the left of the
    more vertical than the left   midline

    For the statement of assertion and reason above state
    which of the following is true

(a) both assertion and reason are true statements and the reason is a correct explanation of the assertion

(b) both assertion and reason are true statements but the reason is *not* a correct explanation of the assertion

(c) the assertion is true, but the reason is a false statement

(d) the assertion is false, but the reason is a true statement

(e) both assertion and reason are false statements

38. Which of the following muscle movements occur during expiration in quiet breathing?

(a) the diaphragm contracts and the intercostal muscles contract

(b) the diaphragm contracts and the intercostal muscles relax

(c) the diaphragm relaxes and the intercostal muscles contract

(d) the diaphragm relaxes and the intercostal muscles relax

39. The mediastinum does *not* contain the

(a) trachea

(b) oesophagus

(c) lung

(d) venae cavae

40. *Assertion*   *Reason*

    During external respira-   the pressure of carbon
    tion oxygen passes from   dioxide in the blood is
    the air to the blood   *because* higher than the pressure
                                        of carbon dioxide in the
                                        alveoli

    For the statement of assertion and reason above state
    which of the following is true

    (a) both assertion and reason are true statements and
        the reason is a correct explanation of the assertion
    (b) both assertion and reason are true statements but
        the reason is not a correct explanation of the
        assertion
    (c) the assertion is true, but the reason is a false
        statement
    (d) the assertion is false, but the reason is a true
        statement
    (e) both assertion and reason are false statements

Chapter 17

41. Vitamin D is necessary in the body for the utilization of

    (a) ergosterol
    (b) calciferol
    (c) calcium
    (d) folic acid

42. What are the end products of normal fat metabolism?

    (a) ketones
    (b) creatinine
    (c) glycerol
    (d) carbon dioxide and water

43. Which of the following vitamins can normally be synthesized in the intestines of an adult?

    (a) vitamin K   (c) vitamin B
    (b) vitamin C   (d) vitamin A

44. Which of the following foods is first-class protein?

    (a) wheat   (c) soya
    (b) milk   (d) beans

45. Which of the following foods is *not* a good source of carbohydrate?

    (a) carrot   (c) parsnip
    (b) wheat   (d) egg

46. Water makes up 60% of the body weight. Most of this water is found

    (a) in the cells   (c) in the blood vessels
    (b) surrounding the cells   (d) in the urinary tract

47. Which one of the following mineral salts might be inadequately provided by the normal diet?

    (a) potassium
    (b) phosphorus
    (c) sodium chloride
    (d) iron

48. Which of the following would require most energy (calories) in the daily diet?

    (a) a boy of 10
    (b) a youth of 17
    (c) a miner of 34
    (d) a housewife of 40

Chapter 18

49. One function of the stomach is to

    (a) activate ptyalin
    (b) convert pepsinogen to pepsin
    (c) form antibodies in infants
    (d) absorb amino acids

50. Which of the following covers the abdominal organs?

    (a) epigastrium
    (b) parietal peritoneum
    (c) visceral peritoneum
    (d) mesentery

51. Which structure attaches the intestine to the posterior abdominal wall?

    (a) mesentery
    (b) visceral peritoneum
    (c) greater omentum
    (d) lesser omentum

52. Vitamin K can be absorbed from the small intestines only in the presence of

    (a) bile
    (b) insulin
    (c) trypsinogen
    (d) amylase

53. Which of the following does *not* help in the digestion of carbohydrate?

    (a) saliva
    (b) gastric juice
    (c) pancreatic juice
    (d) intestinal juice

54. Which of the following is an important factor in the prevention of tooth decay?

    (a) a diet rich in protein
    (b) an adequate supply of vitamin A
    (c) exercising the jaws on crisp food
    (d) an adequate supply of vitamin C

55. Peristalsis is

    (a) a wave of contraction
    (b) a wave of distension
    (c) recoil following distension
    (d) voluntary muscular activity

56. Absorption of food occurs mainly from the

    (a) stomach
    (b) duodenum
    (c) jejunum
    (d) colon

57. The appendix is attached to the

    (a) ileum
    (b) ileocaecal valve
    (c) caecum
    (d) colon

Chapter 19

58. Which of the following is *not* a function of insulin?

    (a) to metabolize carbohydrate
    (b) to metabolize fat
    (c) to allow the entry of glucose into the cells
    (d) to allow the entry of glycogen into the cells

59. Which of the following is *not* a normal function of the adult liver?

    (a) to form urea
    (b) to produce red cells
    (c) to store vitamin D
    (d) to produce heat

60. Failure to produce bile would result in

    (a) inadequate digestion of protein
    (b) scanty urine
    (c) retention of toxic substances
    (d) offensive stools

61. The liver stores

    (a) vitamins B and C
    (b) bile
    (c) iron
    (d) glucose

Chapter 21

62. The function of aldosterone is to

    (a) control the reabsorption of salts by the renal tubules
    (b) control the reabsorption of water by the renal tubules
    (c) constrict the glomerular capillaries
    (d) raise the blood pressure

63. The hormone secreted by the parathyroid glands controls

    (a) the amount of sodium excreted
    (b) the metabolic rate
    (c) the level of calcium in the blood
    (d) the state of mental alertness

64. Tetany may be caused by

    (a) under-secretion of parathyroid hormone
    (b) under-secretion of thyrotrophic hormone
    (c) over-secretion of thyroxine
    (d) over-secretion of parathyroid hormone

65. Thyroid hormone affects all of the following *except*

    (a) water and electrolyte balance
    (b) oxygen consumption
    (c) reproduction
    (d) proper functioning of the nervous system

66. ACTH is secreted by

    (a) the adrenal cortex
    (b) the adrenal medulla
    (c) the hypophysis (pituitary gland)
    (d) the thyroid gland

67. Conditions of stress result in an increase in the activity of the

    (a) hypophysis (pituitary gland)
    (b) adrenal cortex
    (c) adrenal medulla
    (d) thyroid gland

68. Which of the following secretes antidiuretic hormone?

    (a) the anterior lobe of the hypophysis (pituitary gland)
    (b) the posterior lobe of the hypophysis (pituitary gland)
    (c) the adrenal cortex
    (d) the adrenal medulla

Chapter 22

69. Water makes up what percentage of urine?

    (a) 81%
    (b) 86%
    (c) 91%
    (d) 96%

70. Which of the following substances is normally present in the glomerular filtrate?

    (a) thrombocytes
    (b) fibrinogen
    (c) amino acids
    (d) albumin

71. Which function of the kidney is controlled by the antidiuretic hormone?

    (a) reabsorption of water
    (b) reabsorption of salts
    (c) excretion of potassium
    (d) filtration from the glomerulus

72 Fluid is filtered from the glomerulus into the glomerular capsule because

(a) the afferent arteriole is larger than the efferent
(b) the afferent arteriole is smaller than the efferent
(c) the fluid in the renal tubule has a higher osmotic pressure than the blood
(d) the fluid in the renal tubule has a lower osmotic pressure than the blood

Chapter 23

73. There are three layers of tissue (meninges) between the skull and the brain. The cerebrospinal fluid is found between the

(a) arachnoid mater and the pia mater
(b) pia mater and the brain
(c) arachnoid mater and the dura mater
(d) two layers of dura

74. Cerebrospinal fluid is formed mainly in the

(a) subarachnoid space
(b) lateral ventricles
(c) cisterna magna
(d) arachnoid granulations

75. The part of a neuron that conducts impulses away from its cell body is called

    (a) synapse
    (b) afferent fibre
    (c) dendrite
    (d) axon

76. Unconsciousness indicates non-functioning of the

    (a) cerebellum
    (b) cerebral cortex
    (c) hypothalamus
    (d) cerebral nuclei

Chapter 24

77. The arrangement of organs in the middle ear is

    (a) drum, malleus, incus, stapes, oval window
    (b) drum, stapes, incus, malleus, round window
    (c) drum, stapes, incus, malleus, oval window
    (d) drum, malleus, incus, stapes, round window

78. Which part of the ear contains the receptors for hearing?

    (a) middle ear
    (b) semicircular canals
    (c) cochlea
    (d) vestibule

79. Some forms of deafness are associated with loss of balance because both sense organs are

    (a) in the cochlea
    (b) supplied by the same cranial nerve
    (c) in the bony labyrinth
    (d) interpreted in the occipital lobe of the brain

80. In which lobe of the brain does interpretation of sound take place?

    (a) temporal
    (b) parietal
    (c) frontal
    (d) occipital

81. The auditory tube connects the

    (a) nasopharynx and the middle ear
    (b) nasopharynx and the inner ear
    (c) oropharynx and the middle ear
    (d) oropharynx and the inner ear

Chapter 25

82. The nerves causing movement of the eyeball include

    (a) the optic nerve (2nd cranial)
    (b) the facial nerve (7th cranial)
    (c) the trochlear (4th cranial)
    (d) the accessory nerve (11th cranial)

Questions 83, 84 and 85 refer to the diagram of the eye.

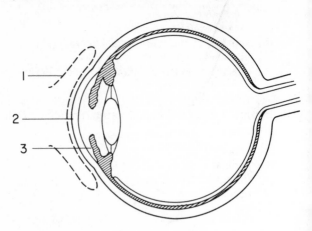

83. The function of the part labelled 1 is to

    (a) lubricate the cornea
    (b) reflect light rays
    (c) protect the underlying structures
    (d) produce lacrimal fluid

84. The part labelled 2 is called

    (a) the conjunctiva
    (b) the cornea
    (c) the choroid
    (d) the sclera

85. The function of the part labelled 3 is to

    (a) give colour to the eye
    (b) control the shape of the lens
    (c) produce aqueous humour
    (d) control the amount of light entering the eye

86. The internal structures of the eye gain their nourishment from

    (a) the aqueous humour
    (b) the vitreous humour
    (c) the internal carotid artery
    (d) the lacrimal fluid

87. The part of the brain responsible for the interpretation of vision is the

    (a) occipital lobe
    (b) temporal lobe
    (c) parietal lobe
    (d) frontal lobe

Chapter 26

88. The skin is able to prevent bacterial entry to the body because of its

    (a) horny outer layer
    (b) good blood supply
    (c) cilia-like action
    (d) natural immunity

89. Which vitamin can be manufactured by the skin?

    (a) C
    (b) D
    (c) E
    (d) K

90. Skin helps in the control of the body temperature because

    (a) it has a rich blood supply
    (b) it has many sensory nerve endings
    (c) it stores quantities of fat
    (d) it has many fine hairs

91. The function of a tactile corpuscle is to

    (a) produce sweat
    (b) cause hairs to stand erect
    (c) secrete sebum
    (d) transmit pressure

Chapter 27

92. The vesicular ovarian (Graafian) follicle produces

    (a) progesterone
    (b) oestrogen
    (c) follicle-stimulating hormone
    (d) luteinizing hormone

93. The corpus luteum produces

    (a) follicle-stimulating hormone
    (b) progesterone
    (c) luteinizing hormone
    (d) oestrogen

94. Where is the ovum most likely to become fertilized?

    (a) in the ovary
    (b) in the uterine (Fallopian) tube
    (c) in the fundus of the uterus
    (d) in the body of the uterus

95. The uterine (Fallopian) tubes are lined with

    (a) mucous membrane
    (b) ciliated epithelium
    (c) fibrous tissue
    (d) pavement epithelium

96. Which of the following is *not* a female sex hormone?

    (a) testosterone
    (b) hexoestrol
    (c) norethisterone
    (d) relaxin

97. The vaginal orifice is partly closed by the

    (a) clitoris
    (b) mons pubis
    (c) hymen
    (d) vestibule

98. The function of the prostate gland is to

    (a) produce spermatozoa
    (b) secrete testosterone
    (c) secrete androgens
    (d) secrete lubricant for the spermatozoa

99. Which of the following produces spermatozoa?

    (a) epididymis
    (b) interstitial cells of testis
    (c) seminal vesicle
    (d) seminiferous tubules

100. Testosterone is secreted by the

    (a) adrenal medulla
    (b) interstitial cells of testis
    (c) seminiferous tubules
    (d) adrenal cortex

Medical Nursing

Chapter 1

1. Match the terms listed in List 1 with the observations in
   List 2

List 1		*List 2*
A pyrexia	1	temperature below 35°C
B hypothermia	2	sudden fall in temperature
C lysis	3	rapid rise in temperature
D rigor		plus shivering
	4	temperature above 37°C
	5	gradual fall in temperature

A	B	C	D

2. Electrolytes are solutions of salts, acids and bases which

   (a) react with glucose to produce an electric charge
   (b) are only found in the cells of the body
   (c) carry an electric charge
   (d) can neutralize a small electric charge

3. Dehydration may be caused by

   (a) reduced intake of food
   (b) drainage from gastrointestinal suction
   (c) intravenous infusion of normal saline
   (d) constipation

4. Match the food constituents in List 1 with their heat
   production (kilojoules (kJ) or kilocalories (kcal/Cal) per
   gram) in List 2

List 1		*List 2*
A protein	1	none
B fats	2	16 kJ (3·8 Cal)
C carbohydrates	3	17 kJ (4 Cal)
D mineral salts	4	30 kJ (9 Cal)
	5	80 kJ (19 Cal)

A	B	C	D

5. Which of the following foods contain no sodium chloride
   and may be used in a 'salt-free' diet?

   (a) meat extracts (e.g. Bovril)
   (b) bread
   (c) milk
   (d) glucose

Chapter 2

6. Which of the following would *not* provide active
   immunity to disease?

   (a) gamma-globulin
   (b) an attack of the disease
   (c) injections of a related organism
   (d) use of a specific vaccine

Chapter 3

7. Match the technical name in List 1 with the description in List 2

	List 1		*List 2*
A	dyspnoea	1	alternating periods of deep breathing with diminished respiration and apnoea
B	apnoea	2	difficulty in breathing
C	orthopnoea	3	inability to breathe unless in the upright position
D	Cheyne-Stokes respiration	4	temporary cessation of breathing
		5	deep sighing breathing

A	B	C	D

8. Which of the following occurs most commonly in chronic bronchitis?

   (a) dry unproductive cough
   (b) excessive sputum
   (c) skin rashes
   (d) pyrexia

9. Which one of the following drugs is *not* used in the treatment of bronchial asthma?

   (a) morphine sulphate
   (b) adrenaline
   (c) hydrocortisone
   (d) ephedrine

10. The amount of oxygen administered to a patient with chronic respiratory disease must be carefully controlled due to the

   (a) possibility of too much being absorbed by the blood
   (b) danger of retention of carbon dioxide
   (c) danger of overstimulation of the heart
   (d) the possibility of damage occurring to the retina of the eyes

11. Lobar pneumonia may be caused by

   1   pneumococcus
   2   aspiration of vomitus postoperatively
   3   virus influenza

   (a) 1 only
   (b) 1 and 2 only
   (c) 1 and 3 only
   (d) 1, 2 and 3

12. Emphysema is caused by

   (a) pus in the pleural cavity
   (b) a chronic cough as in chronic bronchitis
   (c) right-sided heart failure
   (d) coronary thrombosis

13. Which one of the following drugs is *not* used in the treatment of pulmonary tuberculosis?

   (a) PAS
   (b) paracetamol
   (c) INAH
   (d) streptomycin

14. Bronchiectasis is a condition in which there is

    (a) constriction of the main bronchi
    (b) displacement of the bronchial tree
    (c) dilation of bronchioles
    (d) inflammation of the pleura

15. In which of the following conditions is oxygen therapy likely to be used

    1   cor pulmonale
    2   anaemia
    3   asthma

    (a) 1 only
    (b) 3 only
    (c) 1 and 3 only
    (d) 1, 2 and 3

Chapter 4

16. The approximate number of red blood cells which would be considered normal in a woman is

    (a) 2000 000 per mm^3
    (b) 4500 000 per mm^3
    (c) 6000 000 per mm^3
    (d) 12 000 000 per mm^3

17. The erythrocyte sedimentation rate indicates

    (a) the level of white blood cells in the blood
    (b) the level of sodium in the blood
    (c) the level of antibodies in the blood
    (d) the activity of infection in the body

18. Which of the following is *not* found in pernicious (macrocytic) anaemia?

    (a) deficiency of folic acid
    (b) achlorhydria
    (c) disease of the terminal ileum
    (d) lack of the intrinsic factor

19. Vitamin B12 deficiency is *not* likely to occur in

    (a) Crohn's disease
    (b) ulcerative colitis
    (c) vegans (strict vegetarians)
    (d) pernicious anaemia

20. Human blood falls into four main groups. Match the ABO category in List 1 with the statement in List 2

	List 1		*List 2*
A	*A*	1	no A or B antigens in red blood cells but anti-A and anti-B antibodies in plasma
B	*B*		
C	*AB*		
D	*O*	2	A and B antigens in red blood cells but no antibodies in plasma
		3	A antigens in red blood cells and anti-A and B antibodies in plasma
		4	A antigens in red blood cells and anti-B antibodies in plasma
		5	B antigens in red blood cells and anti-A antibodies in plasma

A	B	C	D

Chapter 5

21. Atrial fibrillation is characterized by

    (a) a slow but irregular pulse
    (b) a pulse irregular in force but normal in rate
    (c) an irregular pulse in both time and force
    (d) a weak but regular pulse

The next three questions refer to the case of John Smith who is admitted to the ward with the diagnosis myocardial infarction.

22. Mr Smith's symptoms are likely to include

    1 oedema
    2 dyspnoea
    3 anxiety

    (a) 2 only
    (b) 3 only
    (c) 2 and 3 only
    (d) 1, 2 and 3

23. His immediate treatment is likely to include

    1 rest in bed
    2 morphine sulphate
    3 oxygen

    (a) 1 and 2 only
    (b) 1 and 3 only
    (c) 2 and 3 only
    (d) 1, 2 and 3

24. One purpose of the administration of anticoagulant drugs may be

    (a) to dissolve the clot in the coronary artery
    (b) to prevent spread of the clot in the coronary artery
    (c) to reduce the work of the heart muscle
    (d) to increase peripheral circulation

25. Which one of the following signs and symptoms is most likely to be exhibited by the patient with congestive cardiac failure?

    (a) thirst
    (b) raised blood pressure
    (c) Cheyne–Stokes respiration
    (d) polyuria

26. Which one of the following aspects of nursing care would *not* be adopted in the first 24 hours in hospital for a patient with congestive cardiac failure?

    (a) placing the patient in an upright position in bed
    (b) decreasing sodium in the diet
    (c) frequent attention to pressure areas
    (d) encouraging active movements of the legs

27. Which one of the following drugs would *not* be used for a patient with congestive cardiac failure?

    (a) digoxin
    (b) morphine sulphate
    (c) adrenaline
    (d) Lasix

Chapter 6

28. Match the technical terms in List 1 with the descriptions in List 2

List 1		*List 2*
A dyspepsia	1	vomiting of blood
B hyperchlorhydria	2	absence of acid in stomach
C achlorhydria	3	indigestion
D haematemesis	4	reduced acid in stomach
	5	excess acid in stomach

A	B	C	D

29. Dysphagia may be associated with

   (a) pancreatitis
   (b) congestive cardiac failure
   (c) duodenal ulcer
   (d) achalasia

The following three questions refer to the case of
Mr Jones who has been diagnosed as suffering from a
peptic ulcer.

30. Which one of the following is *not* a symptom of peptic ulceration?

   (a) pain associated with meals
   (b) weight loss
   (c) intolerance of milk
   (d) tiredness

31. Treatment of peptic ulcer is based on

    (a) starvation for 24 hours
    (b) high protein diet
    (c) small regular bland diet
    (d) low calorie diet with vitamin supplements

32. Complications of a peptic ulcer include

    1 haematemesis
    2 pyloric stenosis
    3 oesophageal varices

    (a) 1 and 2 only
    (b) 1 and 3 only
    (c) 2 and 3 only
    (d) 1, 2 and 3

33. Constipation is *not* likely to be caused by

    (a) dietary defects
    (b) worms
    (c) high fluid intake
    (d) lack of exercise

34. Which one of the following is *not* a likely cause of malabsorption of food?

    (a) dislike of taste of the food
    (b) intestinal hurry
    (c) allergy to food constituents
    (d) malformation of part of the small intestine

Chapter 7

35. Jaundice may be caused by

    (a) pancreatitis
    (b) infective hepatitis
    (c) foods which are highly coloured yellow
    (d) anaemia

36. The jaundiced patient is *not* likely to complain of

    (a) skin irritation
    (b) nausea
    (c) urine very pale in colour
    (d) stools very pale in colour

37. Cirrhosis of the liver is commonly caused by

    (a) excess protein in diet
    (b) alcoholism
    (c) diabetes mellitus
    (d) vitamin C deficiency

38. Chronic liver disease is *not* associated with

    (a) abdominal ascites
    (b) spider naevi
    (c) varicose eczema
    (d) jaundice

Chapter 8

39. Simple obesity is usually due to

    (a) hypopituitarism
    (b) hyperthyroidism
    (c) gluttony
    (d) Cushing's syndrome

40. Which of the following will *not* be the cause of rickets?

    (a) lack of sunlight
    (b) dietary deficiency
    (c) chronic lung disease
    (d) longstanding bile duct obstruction

Chapter 9

The following four questions refer to Mary, aged eight years, admitted with acute glomerulonephritis (nephrotic syndrome)

41. Common symptoms of the nephrotic syndrome include

    1 cyanosis
    2 anaemia
    3 albumin in the urine

    (a) 3 only
    (b) 1 and 3 only
    (c) 2 and 3 only
    (d) 1, 2 and 3

42. Mary will be given a high protein diet unless

    (a) protein is lost in the urine
    (b) blood urea is raised
    (c) erythrocyte sedimentation rate is raised
    (d) oedema is increasing

43. When Mary is discharged home her parents will be advised that she should

    (a) avoid crowded places to minimize infection
    (b) have extra games at school to help strengthen the body
    (c) limit her protein intake
    (d) maintain restricted fluid intake

44. Which of the following substances is *not* likely to be found in the urine of a patient with pyelonephritis?

    (a) sugar
    (b) bacteria
    (c) leucocytes
    (d) albumin

45. In the patient who is immobile for a long period (e.g. orthopaedic patient) renal calculi are *not* caused by

    (a) low fluid intake
    (b) decalcification of bones
    (c) urinary infection
    (d) high protein intake

Chapter 10

46. Acute rheumatism (rheumatic fever) in a child is usually associated with

   (a) excessive exercise
   (b) sleeping in a damp bed
   (c) a sore throat
   (d) growing too fast

47. Rheumatoid arthritis is not likely to be treated with

   (a) injections of gold salts (Myocrisin)
   (b) wax baths
   (c) morphine sulphate
   (d) sodium salicylate

Chapter 11

48. Match the terms listed in List 1 with the definitions listed in List 2

List 1		*List 2*
A papule	1	localized oedema of the dermis
B petechiae	2	small raised solid spots
C ecchymoses	3	large purple blotches which do not disappear on pressure
D erythema	4	small haemorrhagic spots
	5	redness of skin, may feel hot to touch

A	B	C	D

49. As a senior nurse on a dermatological ward, which of the following points regarding care of the patients will you *not* make to a new junior nurse?

    (a) most skin conditions are not highly infectious
    (b) these patients are best nursed in cotton rather than woollen blankets
    (c) most patients have got their condition because they did not wash adequately
    (d) the patients frequently find it difficult to sleep

50. Which of the following may be included in the treatment of pruritus?

    (a) hot baths
    (b) sodium bicarbonate solution
    (c) dithranol
    (d) iodine

51. It may be inadvisable to vaccinate a child with infantile eczema because

    (a) the rash of the eczema may hide the vaccination reaction
    (b) the child may show signs of allergic reactions
    (c) the vaccination will be particularly painful
    (d) the vaccination area is likely to develop a secondary infection.

52. Which of the following may be freely consumed by a 16-year-old girl with acne?

    (a) fried foods   (c) cocoa
    (b) chocolate   (d) coffee

53. Psoriasis is frequently associated with

     1   a family history of the condition
     2   a nervous strain
     3   bacterial infection

     (a) 1 and 2 only
     (b) 1 and 3 only
     (c) 2 and 3 only
     (d) 1, 2 and 3

Chapter 12

54. Match the terms listed in List 1 with the definitions in
     List 2

List 1		*List 2*
A paraplegia	1	abnormal sensation, e.g. pins and needles
B paresis	2	uncontrollable shaking
C tremor	3	paralysis of lower part of body
D hyperaesthesia	4	loss of muscle power without paralysis
	5	increased sensibility to heat, cold and pain

A	B	C	D

The following four questions refer to John who is a 20-year-old student who is admitted to the ward following a motor bike accident. He is thought to be unconscious.

55. The observations required to assess level of consciousness would *not* include

   (a) blood pressure recordings
   (b) response to stimuli, e.g. spoken word or touch
   (c) knee reflexes
   (d) urinary output

56. The junior nurse should be told that one of the following signs requires urgent action as it indicates raised intracranial pressure and should therefore be reported immediately

   (a) raised pulse rate and increased respirations
   (b) decreasing pulse rate and rising temperature
   (c) falling temperature and falling blood pressure
   (d) falling blood pressure and falling pulse volume

57. The senior nurse in charge of John should

   (a) maintain silence while attending to him
   (b) avoid touching his eyes or mouth
   (c) teach the junior nurse about his condition while carrying out nursing care
   (d) ensure that his position is changed frequently

58. As John regains consciousness he will *not* be likely to exhibit

    (a) photophobia
    (b) restlessness
    (c) urinary incontinence
    (d) cyanosis

The following three questions refer to Mrs Green aged 76 who is found by her daughter lying on the floor semiconscious and unable to move her left arm and leg. She is admitted to hospital with the diagnosis of cerebral thrombosis (stroke).

59. The reason Mrs Green is unable to move her left arm and leg is that she has sustained damage to the

    (a) cerebellum
    (b) left side of the cerebral cortex
    (c) spinal cord
    (d) right side of the cerebral cortex

60. Which of the following is *not* a main aim of her nursing care?

    (a) maintenance of clear air-way
    (b) keeping the affected limbs at complete rest
    (c) care of pressure areas
    (d) prevention of the development of pneumonia

61. When Mrs Green regains consciousness the main aim of her nursing care will be

    (a) reducing her weight with a low energy diet
    (b) encouraging resumption of normal activity
    (c) ensuring warmth to the affected side
    (d) keeping her quiet so that she will not have another stroke

The following three questions refer to Roger aged 20 years who suffers from grand mal (major) epilepsy

62. The junior nurses should be instructed that when Roger has a fit they should carry out *all but one* of the following

    (a) restrain his arms and legs
    (b) prevent him biting his tongue
    (c) keep his airway clear
    (d) record his actions

63. Which one of the following drugs is *unlikely* to be prescribed?

    (a) sodium phenytoin
    (b) primidone
    (c) paracetamol
    (d) phenobarbitone

64. On discharge Roger is likely to be told that he may indulge in

    (a) swimming
    (b) consumption of alcohol
    (c) riding a bicycle
    (d) dancing

Chapter 13

65. Cybernetic control of a specific hormone such as thyroxine means that it is secreted as a result of

    (a) external administration of its synthetic counterpart
    (b) the blood level of the substance
    (c) emotional excitement
    (d) changes in body temperature

The following three questions relate to Mrs White who has thyrotoxicosis

66. Mrs White has a test to measure her basal metabolic rate (BMR). This is based on

    (a) the amount of food she can eat in 24 hours
    (b) the amount of urine she excretes in 24 hours
    (c) the amount of oxygen she consumes over a given period
    (d) the level of activity she can reach in a given period

67. As a further diagnostic test she is given radio-active iodine (^{131}I) orally. The nurse need *not*

    (a) avoid giving the patient fish prior to the test
    (b) remove the patient's false teeth before giving her the iodine
    (c) nurse the patient behind a lead screen for 24 hours
    (d) ensure that the patient is not having any other drugs containing iodine

68. Mrs White is prescribed antithyroid drugs. These will *not* include

    (a) methylthiouracil
    (b) carbimazole
    (c) potassium perchlorate
    (d) slow K

69. Non-toxic goitre is usually associated with a deficiency of

    (a) salt in the diet
    (b) iodine
    (c) potassium
    (d) phosphorus

70. Mrs Smart is discovered in her house semiconscious. It is not possible to get an ordinary clinical thermometer to register her temperature. It is *unlikely* that the cause of her condition is

    (a) myxoedema
    (b) excessive fluid intake
    (c) a deficiency of protein in her diet
    (d) lack of heating in the house

71. Which of the following is *not* a cause of tetany

    (a) under-activity of the parathyroid glands
    (b) insufficient calcium in the diet
    (c) infection
    (d) inadequate intake of vitamin D

The following seven questions refer to Marion, a 16-year-old girl who is admitted to the ward in a drowsy state. It is likely that she is suffering from diabetes mellitus.

72. Causes of diabetes mellitus do *not* include

    (a) insufficient secretion of insulin by the pancreas
    (b) excessive intake of glucose in food
    (c) resistance of the body to insulin
    (d) disturbance of the pituitary gland

73. Marion is *unlikely* to have complained of

   (a) weight gain
   (b) polyuria
   (c) boils
   (d) thirst

74. The following will *not* be included in the diagnostic tests

   (a) urinalysis
   (b) basal metabolic rate
   (c) blood analysis
   (d) glucose tolerance test

75. The aims of Marion's treatment will *not* include

   (a) controlled intake of carbohydrates
   (b) sufficient food to allow weight maintenance
   (c) sufficient insulin to metabolize glucose intake
   (d) slight restriction of fluid intake

76. Marion is taught that a hypoglycaemic coma is characterized by

   (a) thirst
   (b) disorientation
   (c) breathlessness
   (d) palpitations

77. A junior nurse is to give Marion her 20 units of soluble insulin which she has twice a day. The bottle is labelled 'double strength'. As the nurse in charge of the ward you will tell her to draw up into the syringe

    (a) 0·5 ml
    (b) 1 ml
    (c) 2 ml
    (d) 4 ml

78. Common complications of diabetes mellitus include

    1 retinopathy
    2 peripheral vascular disease
    3 oedema of ankles

    (a) 1 and 2 only
    (b) 1 and 3 only
    (c) 2 and 3 only
    (d) 1, 2 and 3

Chapter 14

79. Infectious diseases are transmitted by

    1 fomites
    2 smells
    3 touch

    (a) 1 and 2 only
    (b) 1 and 3 only
    (c) 2 and 3 only
    (d) 1, 2 and 3

80. In enteric disease the greatest danger to the life of the patient is

    (a) high temperature
    (b) dehydration
    (c) inability to absorb food
    (d) colic

Paediatric Nursing

Chapter 1

1. The average newborn infant can be expected to weigh
   and measure in length approximately

   (a) 2·8 kg and 44 cm
   (b) 3·0 kg and 46 cm
   (c) 3·4 kg and 50 cm
   (d) 3·8 kg and 52 cm

2. The healthy newborn infant can

   (a) react to pain and hunger but cannot see
   (b) hear, see and make reflex movements
   (c) see and react with co-ordinated movements
   (d) make instinctive movements but cannot see

3. Which of the following will the healthy infant *not* be able
   to do at the age of three months?

   (a) lift head off the mattress
   (b) co-ordinate eye movements and fix on objects
   (c) recognize his mother
   (d) be capable of real laughter

4. The average child takes his first steps between

    (a) 8–10 months
    (b) 10–16 months
    (c) 16–18 months
    (d) 18–22 months

5. Which of the following could be described as typical behaviour of a three-month-old baby?

    (a) smiling in response to mother's face and holding head erect
    (a) holding back straight when pulled into a sitting position and recognizing mother
    (c) reaching for and transferring bright objects from one hand to another
    (d) rolling over completely and following bright objects with eyes

6. As a rule the first teeth to erupt at the age of six months are

    (a) two lower central incisors
    (b) two upper central incisors
    (c) two lower lateral incisors
    (d) two upper lateral incisors

7. The number of teeth which the healthy child is likely to have at the age of one year is

    (a) 4–6
    (b) 6–8
    (c) 8–10
    (d) 10–12

8. The ability to walk up a few stairs is normally attained about the age of

    (a) 1 year
    (b) 15 months
    (c) 18 months
    (d) 2 years

9. Which of the following would *not* be considered suitable playthings to encourage the development of a two-year-old child?

    (a) sand and climbing frames
    (b) cuddly teddy or doll
    (c) water and clay
    (d) rattle and beads

10. Which one of the following would give most cause for concern to the nurse?

    (a) a four-year-old child who is not dry at night
    (b) a baby of two months who does not smile
    (c) the child of two and a half years with incomplete dentition
    (d) the child of two years who cannot walk unaided

11. Which of the following can be expected of the *average* child of one year?

    1 pick up small objects
    2 at least 8–10 teeth erupted
    3 build a tower of building bricks

    (a) 1 only
    (b) 2 only
    (c) 1 and 2 only
    (d) 1, 2 and 3

12. Which of the following vaccines can be given orally?

    (a) triple vaccine
    (b) polio vaccine
    (c) tetanus vaccine
    (d) rubella vaccine

13. Against which of the following groups of infectious diseases does the triple vaccine immunize?

    (a) diphtheria, tetanus and pertussis
    (b) tetanus, pertussis and polio
    (c) polio, diphtheria and tetanus
    (d) typhoid, diphtheria and tetanus

Chapter 2

14. In order to avoid the infant swallowing air during bottle feeding the nurse should

    (a) rest the infant after each 30 ml of milk
    (b) allow the infant to take the feed as quickly as possible
    (c) ensure that the bottle teat is always full
    (d) burp the infant before the feed commences

15. Which of the following are reasons why breast feeding is recommended?

    1 it is cheaper
    2 the risk of hypocalcaemic tetany and convulsions is decreased
    3 it establishes a close physical bond between mother and child

    (a) 1 and 2 only
    (b) 1 and 3 only
    (c) 2 and 3 only
    (d) 1, 2 and 3

16. In order to make cow's milk suitable for infants it must be modified. Which of the following changes are necessary?

   1   reduction and breaking up of the amount of casein
   2   reduction in the amount of fat
   3   increase in the amount of carbohydrate
   4   increase in the amount of protein

   (a) 1 only
   (b) 1, 2 and 3 only
   (c) 1, 3 and 4 only
   (d) 2, 3 and 4 only

17. *Assertion*   *Reason*
    It is advisable to give   iron is stored in the
    all premature infants   liver of the fetus
    iron supplements   *because*   from the 13th to 40th
                                         week of gestation

    With reference to the statement above which of the following is true?

    (a) both assertion and reason are true statements and the reason is a correct explanation of the assertion
    (b) both assertion and reason are true statements but the reason is not a correct explanation of the assertion
    (c) the assertion is true, but the reason is a false statement
    (d) the assertion is false, but the reason is a true statement
    (e) both assertion and reason are false statements

Chapters 3 and 4

18. *Assertion*

    The newborn infant has difficulty in maintaining a stable body temperature

    because

    Reason

    the heat regulating centre is immature and the body surface area is large in proportion to weight

    With reference to the statement above which of the following is true?

    (a) both assertion and reason are true statements and the reason is a correct explanation of the assertion
    (b) both assertion and reason are true statements but the reason is not a correct explanation of the assertion
    (c) the assertion is true but the reason is a false statement
    (d) the assertion is false but the reason is a true statement
    (e) both assertion and reason are false statements

19. Which of the following features does the premature infant possess

    1 large head in comparison to body size
    2 wrinkled skin and thin limbs
    3 short soft finger and toe nails

    (a) 1 only
    (b) 1 and 2 only
    (c) 1, 2 and 3
    (d) 2 only

20. The stools of infants fed on any type of cow's milk compared to breast fed infants are likely to be

    (a) dark yellow and more bulky
    (b) dark yellow and looser
    (c) pale yellow, bulky and more formed
    (d) pale yellow, soft and less formed

21. To prevent hypoglycaemia in the newborn low-birth-weight infant which of the following would the nurse expect as part of the infant's care?

    1 feeding should commence early
    2 regular estimations of blood sugar levels should be made
    3 undue exertion of the infant should be avoided

    (a) 1 only
    (b) 1 and 2 only
    (c) 2 and 3 only
    (d) 1, 2 and 3

22. The low-birth-weight infant's feeding requirements at the age of two weeks are (for every 200 ml/kg/day)

    (a) 110–130 calories (462–546 J)
    (b) 130–150 calories (546–620 J)
    (c) 150–160 calories (620–672 J)
    (d) 160–170 calories (672–722 J)

Chapter 5

23. Which one of the following should the nurse report to the paediatrician?

    (a) stork beak marks
    (b) milia on the face
    (c) enlarged breasts
    (d) dried umbilical cord

24. A mother whose baby has a cavernous naevus (strawberry mark) should be told that the naevus will

    (a) remain the same size for a while, then disappear
    (b) become darker and smaller
    (c) remain the same
    (d) grow larger then disappear

25. *Assertion*   *Reason*
    Physiological jaundice   the liver is unable
    occurs in 50% of newborn   *because* to excrete bilirubin
    infants

    With reference to the statement above, which of the
    following is true?

    (a) both assertion and reason are true statements and
         the reason is a correct explanation of the assertion
    (b) both assertion and reason are true statements but
         the reason is not a correct explanation of the
         assertion
    (c) the assertion is true but the reason is a false
         statement
    (d) the assertion is false but the reason is a true
         statement
    (e) both assertion and reason are false statements

26. A maternal history of hydramnios in pregnancy should
    alert the nurse to the possibility of the following in the
    newborn infant

    1   tracheo-oesophageal fistula
    2   duodenal obstruction
    3   anal stenosis

    (a) 1 only
    (b) 1 and 2 only
    (c) 1 and 3 only
    (d) 1, 2 and 3

27. Which one of the following would lead the nurse to suspect tracheo-oesophageal fistula in the newborn?

    (a) frequent harsh coughing attacks
    (b) cyanosis and refusal to take feeds
    (c) coughing and choking with feeding
    (d) respiratory distress with cyanosis

28. In patent ductus arteriosus there is an abnormal opening between the

    (a) right and left atria
    (b) right ventricle and aorta
    (c) aorta and pulmonary artery
    (d) right and left ventricles

29. The administration of excess oxygen to a premature infant may result in

    (a) retrolental fibroplasia
    (b) spasticity
    (c) nystagmus
    (d) respiratory distress

Chapter 6

30. Which of the following behaviour patterns might be expected from children under the age of five years who are admitted to hospital?

    1   regression to a former stage of development
    2   become very quiet, co-operative and good
    3   do not gain weight and may fail to thrive

    (a) 1 only
    (b) 3 only
    (c) 1 and 2 only
    (d) 1, 2 and 3

31. Accompanied by his mother, a child aged two years is admitted to the children's ward sucking a dummy. What course of action should you take?

    (a) remove the dummy and give it to his mother
    (b) ignore the situation and let the child keep the dummy
    (c) take the dummy away and give the child a toy
    (d) let the child keep the dummy for the time being, then remove when he is asleep

32. In the children's ward it is desirable to have

    (a) visiting every afternoon
    (b) no visiting immediately after operation or treatments
    (c) visiting only by father or mother
    (d) completely unrestricted visiting

Chapter 8

33. The average respiration rate of the child aged one year is (per minute)

    (a) 18–20
    (b) 20–24
    (c) 24–30
    (d) 30–40

34. Which of the following are likely to precipitate an attack of asthma in the susceptible child?

    1 over-exertion
    2 allergy
    3 infection

    (a) 1 only
    (b) 1 and 3 only
    (c) 2 and 3 only
    (d) 1, 2 and 3

Chapter 9

35. Acute laryngotracheitis is most commonly caused by

    (a) viral infection of the upper respiratory tract
    (b) an allergic reaction in the larynx
    (c) bacterial infection of the upper respiratory tract
    (d) obstruction of the trachea

36. During the immediate postoperative period following tonsillectomy which of the following would cause the nurse to suspect haemorrhage?

    1   restlessness
    2   rising pulse rate
    3   repeated swallowing
    4   constricted pupils

    (a) 1 and 2 only
    (b) 1, 2 and 3 only
    (c) 2 and 3 only
    (d) 2, 3 and 4 only

The next two questions refer to James aged three months who has been admitted for repair of a cleft lip.

37. Which of the following would indicate to the surgeon postponement of the operation?

    (a) haemoglobin level of 70 mg/100 ml
    (b) weight of 5·5 kg
    (c) Rhesus-negative blood group
    (d) James is being breast-fed

38. Before repair of the cleft lip, the nurse would ensure that James is fed by

    (a) bottle and teat
    (b) Belcroy feeder
    (c) a bent teaspoon
    (d) feeding cup

Chapter 10

The next two questions refer to Ruth, four months old
and in cardiac failure.

39. Which of the following would best describe her
    condition?

    1   irritable cough, breathless and sweating
    2   eager for feeds and failing to gain weight
    3   restless, anorexic and difficult to feed

    (a) 1 only
    (b) 1 and 2 only
    (c) 1 and 3 only
    (d) 2 and 3 only

40. You should nurse Ruth in an upright position in order to

    (a) facilitate feeding
    (b) enable Ruth to look around the ward
    (c) reduce abdominal distension
    (d) facilitate breathing and assist lung expansion

41. On some occasions hypothermia is used in open heart
    surgery in order to

    (a) reduce the metabolism and body oxygen
         requirements
    (b) minimize postoperative complications
    (c) maintain normal respiration during anaesthesia
    (d) reduce cardiac activity

42. During the immediate postoperative period which of the following would you *not* need to do in your care of a patient who has undergone cardiac surgery?

    (a) observe that the fluid in the chest drainage tubes oscillates between respirations
    (b) measure the blood loss in the drainage bottles every half hour
    (c) release urinary catheter frequently and regularly measure urine output
    (d) keep the child covered with a light blanket

Chapter 11

43. Sally aged seven years has rheumatic fever and will require considerable nursing care whilst on complete bed rest. The nurse should therefore

    1 give a bed bath when appropriate
    2 feed Sally with an interesting diet
    3 sit her up, supported with several pillows
    4 provide her with suitable play material

    (a) 1, 3 and 4 only
    (b) 1, 2 and 3 only
    (c) 1, 2, 3 and 4
    (d) 2, 3 and 4 only

44. The pulse rate in rheumatic fever can best be described as

    (a) rapid both awake and sleeping
    (b) slow whilst awake, rapid during sleep
    (c) rapid whilst awake, slow during sleep
    (d) normal whilst awake and sleep

Chapter 12

45. As an inherited disease sickle-cell anaemia is most common amongst the descendants of

    (a) Negroes
    (b) Semitic peoples
    (c) Mediterranean races
    (d) Asians

46. The diet of a child with iron deficiency anaemia should include

    1 eggs
    2 chocolate
    3 wholemeal bread
    4 potatoes

    (a) 1, 2 and 3 only
    (b) 1, 3 and 4 only
    (c) 1, 2, 3 and 4
    (d) 2, 3 and 4 only

47. Bone marrow puncture may be performed in the investigation of blood disorders. The site most commonly used in a child aged three years would be

    (a) sternum
    (b) iliac crest
    (c) tibial shaft
    (d) radius

48. Methotrexate and 6-mercaptopurine are commonly used in the treatment of leukaemia. Which of the following would alert the nurse to the possibility of drug toxicity?

    1 mouth ulcers and secondary infection
    2 vomiting and constipation
    3 hair loss and alopecia
    4 nystagmus and blurred vision

    (a) 1 only
    (b) 1 and 4 only
    (c) 1, 2 and 3 only
    (d) 1, 2, 3 and 4

49. Haemophilia is a bleeding disease transmitted by the

    (a) father to sons
    (b) mother to sons
    (c) father to daughters
    (d) mother to daughters

Chapter 13

50. Which of the following would be expected of the infant with pyloric stenosis?

    (a) anaemia
    (b) metabolic alkalosis
    (c) vitamin deficiency
    (d) hypothermia

51. The stools of the infant with pyloric stenosis can be described as

    (a) soft, yellow and frequent
    (b) normal consistency but infrequent
    (c) small, green and seldom
    (d) large, bulky and offensive

52. Which of the following would you expect to find in an infant with gastroenteritis?

    1   body temperature 39·4°C and tachycardia
    2   depressed fontanelle, skin dry and elastic
    3   serum chlorides 98–106 mEq/litre

    (a) 2 only
    (b) 1 and 2 only
    (c) 2 and 3 only
    (d) 1, 2 and 3

53. *Assertion*   *Reason*
    Intussusception results in   a piece of bowel has
    intestinal obstruction   *because*   invaginated into the
                                          bowel beyond

    With reference to the statement above which of the
    following is true?

    (a) both assertion and reason are true statements and
         the reason is a correct explanation of the assertion
    (b) both assertion and reason are true statements but
         the reason is not a correct explanation of the
         assertion
    (c) the assertion is true but the reason is a false
         statement
    (d) the assertion is false but the reason is a true
         statement
    (e) both assertion and reason are false statements

54. Which of the following would confirm threadworm
    infestation?

    (a) serum sample
    (b) Sellotape test
    (c) visual examination of the stools
    (d) skin test

55. Which of the following features are characteristically
    found in Hirschsprung's disease?

    1   thin ribbon-like stools
    2   borborygmus and distended abdomen
    3   anorexia and vomiting

    (a) 1 only
    (b) 1 and 2 only
    (c) 2 and 3 only
    (d) 1, 2 and 3

56. The care of a child prior to Swenson's operation would include

    1   rectal washouts
    2   blood grouping and cross matching
    3   barium meal

    (a) 1 and 3 only
    (b) 2 only
    (c) 1 and 2 only
    (d) 1, 2 and 3

Chapter 14

57. Which of the following diseases is the Guthrie test used to detect?

    (a) coeliac disease
    (b) phenylketonuria
    (c) maple syrup disease
    (d) cystic fibrosis

58. The successful treatment of phenylketonuria depends on

    (a) maintaining plasma phenylalanine levels below
        5 mg/100 ml
    (b) keeping the Phenistix test negative
    (c) balancing phenylalanine intake with urinary output
    (d) eliminating phenylalanine from the diet

The next three questions refer to Ann, age two years, who has been admitted with a chest infection

59. Which of the following should alert the nurse to the possibility of cystic fibrosis?

    1 bulky, offensive stools
    2 failure to thrive
    3 strong musty smelling urine

    (a) 1 only
    (b) 2 only
    (c) 2 and 3 only
    (d) 1 and 2 only

60. The diagnosis of cystic fibrosis has been made, and in Ann's treatment pancreatic preparations must be given; the best times for these are

    (a) before meals
    (b) with meals
    (c) after meals
    (d) at four-hourly intervals during the day

61. Which of the following should be given to Ann as supplements to her diet?

    (a) water-soluble vitamins
    (b) fat-soluble vitamins
    (c) ferrous sulphate
    (d) ketovite

62. A gluten-free diet should exclude all preparations containing

    (a) barley and corn
    (b) rye and oats
    (c) wheat and rye
    (d) maize and wheat

Chapter 15

63. Which of the following would lead the nurse to suspect hypothyroidism in the young infant?

    (a) the skin is yellow, coarse and dry with bradycardia and hypothermia
    (b) the baby is fat, oedematous and breathless
    (c) the mother tells you that she has had a thyroidectomy
    (d) there is a reluctance to feed, sore buttocks and diarrhoea

64. Initially with thyroid treatment the infant with hypothyroidism will

    1   appear more alert and active
    2   lose weight
    3   increase body temperature

    (a) 1 only
    (b) 1 and 3 only
    (c) 2 and 3 only
    (d) 1, 2 and 3

65. Which of the following would alert the nurse to the possibility of diabetes mellitus in a child aged six years?

    (a) obesity
    (b) headaches
    (c) excessive hunger
    (d) enuresis of sudden onset

66. The diabetic child is taught to vary the injection site for insulin because

    (a) tissue necrosis may occur
    (b) fat atrophy may develop
    (c) it is less painful
    (d) it is easier for the child to manage

Chapter 16

67. John aged eight years has been admitted with nephritis. Which of the following would you expect to find associated with his condition?

    1 vomiting and headaches
    2 weight loss of sudden onset
    3 hypertension and haematuria

    (a) 3 only
    (b) 1 and 2 only
    (c) 1 and 3 only
    (d) 1, 2 and 3

Chapter 17

68. Persistent nocturnal enuresis is most frequently associated with

    (a) behavioural disorders
    (b) urinary tract infections
    (c) congenital abnormalities of the urinary tract
    (d) encopresis

69. The most common organism causing meningitis in the neonatal period is

    (a) *Haemophilus influenzae*
    (b) *Escherichia coli*
    (c) meningococcus
    (d) tubercle bacillus

70. Mental handicap may be caused by

    1 genetic factors
    2 antenatal infection or birth injury
    3 postnatal infection or trauma

    (a) 1 only
    (b) 1 and 3 only
    (c) 2 and 3 only
    (d) 1, 2 and 3

71. *Assertion*   *because*   *Reason*
    Parents of mentally handicapped children need to encourage more, not less, normal childhood activities such as play and nursery rhymes   these children do not learn through normal schooling

    With reference to the above statement which of the following is true?

    (a) both assertion and reason are true statements and the reason is a correct explanation of the assertion
    (b) both assertion and reason are true statements but the reason is not a correct explanation of the assertion
    (c) the assertion is true but the reason is a false statement
    (d) the assertion is false but the reason is a true statement
    (e) both assertion and reason are false statements

Chapter 18

72. Infantile eczema is

    (a) of unknown cause
    (b) an allergic response
    (c) a familial condition
    (d) of metabolic origin

73. The nursing care for a child with eczema should be designed to

    1   keep him cool and suitably occupied
    2   give him the appropriate diet and soothing baths
    3   keep isolated to avoid risk of infection

    (a) 1 only
    (b) 1 and 2 only
    (c) 2 and 3 only
    (d) 1, 2 and 3

Chapter 19

74. Which of the following would alert the nurse to the possibility of congenital dislocation of the hip in the neonate?

    1   positive Ortolani's sign
    2   well-developed gluteal muscles
    3   tendency for the infant to roll onto one side

    (a) 1 only
    (b) 1 and 3 only
    (c) 2 and 3 only
    (d) 1, 2 and 3

75. The success of treatment for talipes equinovarus depends on

    1   commencing treatment within 36 hours of birth
    2   frequent manipulation
    3   splinting the foot in an over-corrected position

    (a) 1 only
    (b) 2 only
    (c) 1 and 3 only
    (d) 1, 2 and 3

Chapter 21

76. Koplik's spots are found in the prodromal stages of

    (a) chicken pox
    (b) rubella
    (c) measles
    (d) scarlet fever

77. Which of the following infectious diseases is *not* notifiable?

    (a) measles
    (b) diphtheria
    (c) scarlet fever
    (d) rubella

78. Children with chicken pox should be kept segregated until

    (a) all the scabs have fallen off
    (b) all the scabs are dry
    (c) the temperature has returned to normal
    (d) 2–3 days after the rash has disappeared

79. Which of the following groups should be given Bacille
    Calmette–Guerin (BCG) inoculation?

    (a) all children under the age of five years
    (b) all children of school leaving age
    (c) children of school leaving age who are Mantoux
        positive
    (d) infants with a close relative who has TB

Chapter 22

80. Alan aged six years has been admitted with 15% full
    thickness burns. During the first 48 hours a reduction of
    urine output is reported, what should this alert the nurse
    to?

    1   inadequate fluid replacement
    2   impending renal failure
    3   urinary tract infection

    (a) 1 only
    (b) 1 and 2 only
    (c) 2 and 3 only
    (d) 1, 2 and 3

Surgical Nursing

Chapter 1

1. The safest method of sterilizing cystoscopes is

   (a) autoclaving
   (b) pasteurization
   (c) hot dry air
   (d) flaming

Chapter 2

2. Match up the type of wound in List 1 with the possible causation in List 2

List 1		*List 2*
A incised	1	gun shot
B lacerated	2	knife slash
C punctured	3	shell fragment
	4	truncheon blow

A	B	C

3. Shock arising due to loss of fluid from the body, such as an arterial haemorrhage is called

   (a) neurogenic
   (b) oligaemic
   (c) vasomotor
   (d) toxaemic

4. An arterial haemorrhage can be recognized from the fact
   that the blood normally

   (a) spurts from the proximal side of the wound
   (b) spurts from the distal side of the wound
   (c) wells up evenly from the proximal side of the wound
   (d) wells up evenly from the distal side of the wound

5. Haemorrhage is suspected when

   (a) the temperature of the patient's body rises
   (b) the pulse rate increases and the blood pressure falls
   (c) the pulse rate falls and the blood pressure rises
   (d) pulse rate drops and the respiratory rate rises

6. Air hunger developing in a shocked patient indicates

   (a) haemorrhage
   (b) myocardial infarction
   (c) hypoproteinaemia
   (d) heart failure

7. Haematemesis is always caused by

   (a) perforation of the stomach wall caused by a gastric
       ulcer
   (b) erosion of a blood vessel in the stomach
   (c) oesophageal varices
   (d) generalized acute gastritis

8. Match the routes of fluid loss from the body in List 1 with the volumes lost per day in List 2

List 1		*List 2*
A expiration	1	150 ml
B perspiration	2	350 ml
C in urine	3	500 ml
D in faeces	4	1500 ml
	5	2500 ml

A	B	C	D

9. A young conscious patient is receiving intravenous fluids and develops a 'bubbly cough', rising pulse rate and dyspnoea. Which of the following courses of action will you and the doctor take first?

   (a) obtain a specimen of sputum for culture and sensitivity
   (b) slow down or stop the intravenous fluids
   (c) administer oxygen
   (d) prepare for a chest aspiration

10. A Rhesus-negative woman is not normally given a transfusion of Rhesus-positive blood because it would

   (a) increase the risk of emboli formation
   (b) cause painful venous spasm
   (c) cause anti-D to form in her blood
   (d) cause her blood to become Rhesus-positive

11. Under what conditions should blood be stored?

    (a) at a temperature of 24°C
    (b) in a cool dark cupboard
    (c) in a deep-freezer
    (d) at a temperature of 4°C

12. Which of the following agglutinins are found in group AB blood?

    (a) agglutinin a only
    (b) agglutinin b only
    (c) agglutinins a and b
    (d) no agglutinins at all

Chapter 3

13. Septicaemia is a condition where

    (a) there is formation of secondary abscesses due to the presence of septic foci
    (b) transient bacteria are present in the blood stream
    (c) actively multiplying bacteria are present in the blood stream
    (d) *Staphylococcus aureus* is present in the cellular tissues

14. If a farmer who has sustained a crushed limb when his tractor fell on top of him, develops intense wound pain, discoloration of tissues, a foul-smelling discharge from the wound and is obviously very toxic, then which of the following conditions must be suspected?

    (a) tetanus
    (b) gas gangrene
    (c) botulism
    (d) undulant fever

Chapter 4

15. A patient has been admitted with burns involving the whole of the trunk. What percentage of the body surface area is involved?

    (a) 9%
    (b) 18%
    (c) 36%
    (d) 50%

16. The haematocrit (PCV) of a normally healthy adult is

    (a) 25%
    (b) 45%
    (c) 65%
    (d) 85%

17. Which of the following intravenous fluids may be of most value in the emergency treatment of a severely burnt patient?

    (a) packed cells
    (b) normal saline
    (c) dextran
    (d) 5% glucose

18. Plasma is most likely to be used in the treatment of

    (a) burns
    (b) haemophilia
    (c) chronic anaemia
    (d) defibrination syndrome

19. A burnt limb should be positioned

    (a) above the level of the trunk and extended
    (b) below the level of the trunk and extended
    (c) above the level of the trunk and flexed
    (d) below the level of the trunk and flexed

Chapter 5

20. Which type of traction is being used when a Steinmann's pin has been introduced?

    (a) skull traction
    (b) skin traction
    (c) pulp traction
    (d) skeletal traction

21. Rising intracranial pressure is suspected when

    (a) temperature rises and blood pressure falls
    (b) pulse rate increases and blood pressure falls
    (c) pulse rate falls and blood pressure rises
    (d) temperature and pulse rate drop

22. A patient with Colles' fracture immobilized in plaster of Paris must be encouraged to

    (a) move fingers and shoulders on the same day
    (b) rest the fingers and shoulders for a week
    (c) move only shoulders
    (d) move only fingers

23. Which of the following may be used to replace the femoral head?

    (a) Austin Moore prosthesis
    (b) McLaughlin pin and plate
    (c) Steinmann's pin
    (d) Kunchner nail

24. The most common type of fractured patella, such as occurs when a person's knee strikes the dash board in a car accident, is called

    (a) impacted
    (b) transverse
    (c) comminuted
    (d) spiral

Chapter 6

25. Which of the following is *not* characteristic of a malignant tumour?

    (a) it is enclosed in a capsule of fibrous tissue
    (b) many cells undergoing active mitosis can be seen within the tumour
    (c) the tumour tends to spread rapidly
    (d) it is recognized as scirrhous on histology

26. A melanotic tumour is one which

   (a) develops in the glands of the breast
   (b) becomes pigmented; black or dark brown in colour
   (c) is a round smooth tumour composed of fat cells
   (d) develops in the epithelial cells of the stomach

Chapter 7

27. The route by which the anaesthetic thiopentone sodium (Pentothal) is administered is

   (a) intravenous
   (b) intrathecal
   (c) intra-arterial
   (d) intramuscular

28. The anaesthetic agent Trilene is administered

   (a) intravenously
   (b) orally
   (c) by inhalation
   (d) intrathecally

29. Tubocurarine (Tubarine) is a

    (a) muscle relaxant
    (b) respiratory stimulant
    (c) local anaesthetic
    (d) cardiac stimulant

30. Intravenous suxamethonium (Scoline) is given to a patient in the anaesthetic room to cause

    (a) increased depth of coma
    (b) muscular relaxation
    (c) reduction of secretions
    (d) return to consciousness

31. Indicate from the following list the correct sequence of action to be taken if a patient has a cardiac arrest while you are on the ward with a junior nurse at night

    (a) instruct your junior to obtain medical aid
    (b) commence external heart massage
    (c) clear the patients airway
    (d) commence mouth to mouth respiration (or use an Ambubag) and give oxygen

1	2	3	4

Chapter 8

32. 'Consent for operation' forms should be signed by

    (a) the patient only
    (b) the patient and his next of kin only
    (c) the patient and the admitting doctor
    (d) the ward sister and the patient

33. Deep vein thrombosis of the calf can be treated by

    (a) vitamin K
    (b) antibiotic therapy
    (c) low protein diet
    (d) anticoagulant therapy

Chapter 9

34. Carcinoma of the tongue is most likely to be treated by

    (a) implant of radium needles
    (b) stilboestrol by mouth
    (c) hypophysectomy
    (d) radio-active iodine

35. Postoperative tetany may be due to

    (a) damage to the recurrent laryngeal nerve
    (b) removal or damage to the parathyroid glands
    (c) removal of too much of the thyroid gland
    (d) release of a large volume of thyroxine into the blood from the thyroid gland

36. The physiological dead space is normally described as

    (a) air in the respiratory passages that is not directly involved in gaseous exchange
    (b) the air that is forced out of the lungs when a corpse is moved from side to side
    (c) the air that is contained in the tubing between the patient and a mechanical ventilator
    (d) the air left in the lungs after a quiet expiration

37. Which of the following tracheostomy tubes has an optional speaking valve?

    (a) Durham's lobster tailed
    (b) Negus
    (c) Parker's
    (d) cuffed Radcliffe

38. Which of the following tracheostomy tubes may be used if positive pressure ventilation is required?

    (a) Negus
    (b) Durham's lobster tail
    (c) cuffed Radcliffe
    (d) Chevalier Jackson

39. Complications of tracheostomy include

    1 infection of the chest
    2 surgical emphysema
    3 wound sepsis

    (a) 1 and 2 only
    (b) 1 and 3 only
    (d) 2 and 3 only
    (d) 1, 2 and 3

40. Surgical emphysema is described as

    (a) reduced lung function due to overdistension of the alveoli
    (b) a collection of pus in the lungs
    (c) air in the subcutaneous tissue
    (d) a collection of pus between muscle fibres

Chapter 10

41. Which of the following would cause you to believe that damage to the oesophagus had occurred during an oesophagoscopy?

    1 vomiting of bile-stained fluid
    2 on examination with X-rays air and fluid recognized in the pleural cavities
    3 rigidity in the upper abdominal muscles, pain and shock

    (a) 1 and 2 only
    (b) 1 and 3 only
    (c) 2 and 3 only
    (d) 1, 2 and 3

42. Before an oesophagoscopy a local anaesthetic is used. Indicate which of the following statements concerning after care are correct

    1 the patient is usually allowed out of bed on the same day
    2 decicain lozenges 25 or 60 mg are given every 3 hours
    3 food and fluids are withheld until the effects of the local anaesthetic have worn off

    (a) 1 and 2 only
    (b) 1 and 3 only
    (c) 2 and 3 only
    (d) 1, 2 and 3

43. Carcinoma of the oesophagus occurs most commonly amongst

    (a) men in early middle age
    (b) men aged 50 to 70 years
    (c) women in early middle age
    (d) women aged 50 to 70 years

Chapter 11

44. Match up the definitions in List 1 and the name of the lung volume in List 2

List 1		*List 2*
A normal volume of air breathed in and out in one respiration	1	vital capacity
B volume of air in the lungs at the end of each quiet expiration	2	tidal volume
C the maximum possible inspiration and expiration	3	tidal volume plus inspiratory reserve volume
D the volume of air taken in at the greatest inspiratory effort	4	residual volume
	5	functional residual capacity

A	B	C	D

45. Which of the following characteristics apply to a two-year-old child with Fallot's tetralogy?

    1 poor physical development
    2 sits in a squatting position
    3 anaemia

    (a) 1 and 2 only
    (b) 1 and 3 only
    (c) 2 and 3 only
    (d) 1, 2 and 3

46. Fallot's tetralogy is due to

    (a) an infection at birth
    (b) anoxia at birth
    (c) neoplasm
    (d) congenital malformation

47. Which of the following conditions is *not* classified as an acyanotic defect?

    (a) patent ductus arteriosus
    (b) Fallot's tetralogy
    (c) coarctation of aorta
    (d) atrial septal defect

Chapter 12

48. A patient's varicose vein has ruptured and there is a profuse haemorrhage. Which of the following should be done?

    1 apply a tourniquet direct to the thigh
    2 apply direct pressure to the bleeding point
    3 raise the leg

    (a) 1 and 2 only
    (b) 1 and 3 only
    (c) 2 and 3 only
    (d) 1, 2 and 3

49. Which of the following instructions would be given to a patient with varicose ulcers?

   1   avoid standing still in one position
   2   sleep with the foot of the bed raised
   3   do not sit too close to the fire

   (a) 1 and 2 only
   (b) 1 and 3 only
   (c) 2 and 3 only
   (d) 1, 2 and 3

Chapter 13

50. A recent retraction or inversion of the nipple in a 50-year-old woman is likely to be due to

   (a) abscess
   (b) adenoma
   (c) cyst
   (d) a breast cancer

Chapter 14

51. A patient develops the following signs and symptoms 48 hours following surgery

   1   progressive (faecal) vomiting
   2   marked abdominal distension
   3   absence of bowel sounds

   What is likely to be wrong with this patient?

   (a) impaction of faeces
   (b) paralytic ileus
   (c) alkalosis
   (d) early peritonitis

52. A patient is admitted and has severe abdominal pain; his abdomen is rigid and board-like. His pulse rate is rapid and abdominal movements do not take place on respiration. What is the most probable diagnosis?

    (a) intestinal obstruction
    (b) bronchial pneumonia
    (c) acute peritonitis
    (d) ruptured kidney

53. Which of the following situations would be considered abnormal when aspirating a Ryles/Levin tube?

    1 fresh blood aspirated 24 hours following gastric surgery
    2 increasing volumes of aspirate following gastric surgery
    3 air bubbling in and out of the tube on respiration

    (a) 1 and 2 only
    (b) 1 and 3 only
    (c) 2 and 3 only
    (d) 1, 2 and 3

Chapter 15

54. Which type of acid is produced in the stomach?

    (a) hydrochloric
    (b) sulphuric
    (c) phosphoric
    (d) nitric

55. A vagotomy is performed to

    (a) speed up the passage of food through the stomach
    (b) decrease the acid secretion of the stomach
    (c) decrease the movement of the stomach
    (d) increase the acid secretion of the stomach

56. Projectile vomiting developing in a previously healthy baby of three to four weeks of age suggests

    (a) intussusception
    (b) volvulus
    (c) pyloric stenosis
    (d) paralytic ileus

Chapter 16

57. Match up the sites of incision in List 1 with the most likely operations in List 2

List 1		*List 2*
A right iliac fossa	1	prostatectomy
B mid line	2	nephrectomy
C loin above iliac crest	3	appendicectomy
D suprapubic	4	partial gastrectomy
	5	left lower lobectomy

A	B	C	D

58. The passage of blood-stained mucus from the rectum of a child that draws up its legs and screams because of the 'colicky' pain may indicate

    (a) volvulus
    (b) pyloric stenosis
    (c) intussusception
    (d) carcinoma in large bowel

59. Indicate which one of the following conditions may be treated by means of an ileostomy

    (a) haematemesis
    (b) starvation due to inoperable carcinoma
    (c) ulcerative colitis
    (d) pyloric stenosis

Chapter 17

60. Patients with surgical jaundice have

    (a) a blocked bile duct
    (b) hepatitis
    (c) excessive haemolysis
    (d) pernicious anaemia

61. Match up the operations in List 1 with its description in List 2

List 1		*List 2*
A cholecystectomy	1	opening common bile duct to remove stone and insert drain
B cholecystostomy		
C cholecystgastrostomy	2	opening gall bladder to remove stone and insert drain
D choledochotomy		
	3	dissection of inflamed gall bladder from liver
	4	removal of gall bladder
	5	anastamosis of gall bladder to stomach

A	B	C	D

62. Which of the following vitamins is required to allow the liver to produce prothrombin?

    (a) B1
    (b) B12
    (c) E
    (d) K

63. Kehr's 'T' drainage tubes are used to provide drainage following operations on

    (a) any part of the abdomen
    (b) the common bile duct
    (c) the urinary bladder
    (d) the small bowel

64. Excision of part of the pancreas and reconstruction of the bile ducts is called

    (a) Ramstedt's operation
    (b) Whipple's operation
    (c) Wertheim's operation
    (d) choledochotomy

65. Vitamin K may be prescribed and administered to a jaundiced patient before surgery on the biliary tract in order to

    (a) increase reabsorption of sodium in the kidney tubule
    (b) reduce the risk of bleeding
    (c) reduce the risk of thrombus formation
    (d) increase the flow of bile into the duodenum

Chapter 18

66. Match the types of hernia in List 1 with the description in List 2

List 1		*List 2*
A inguinal	1	common in babies and elderly fat women
B ventral	2	sited above Poupart's ligament
C hiatus	3	protruding up through the diaphragm
D umbilical	4	arising through a healed operation wound
	5	twisting of the bowel on itself

A	B	C	D

Chapter 19

67. A track leading from the skin near the anus to part of the anal canal or rectum is called a(n)

    (a) pilonidal sinus
    (b) fistula-in-ano
    (c) ischiorectal abscess
    (d) fissure-in-ano

68. An infant who fails to pass meconium during the first 24 hours after birth may have

    (a) volvulus of the descending colon
    (b) mesenteric thrombosis
    (c) imperforate anus
    (d) imperforate hymen

69. A neighbour complains to you of a sense of fullness in the rectum after defaecation and alternating constipation and diarrhoea. What would they cause you to suspect?

    (a) internal haemorrhoids
    (b) ulcerative colitis
    (c) carcinoma of the rectum
    (d) fistula-in-ano

70. A male patient has still not passed urine 18 hours following a haemorrhoidectomy. His bladder is obviously distended but his general condition is satisfactory. Which *one* of the following courses of action can you take without medical permission?

    (a) catheterize the patient
    (b) allow him to stand at the side of the bed to micturate
    (c) sit him in a hot bath
    (d) administer a diuretic

Chapter 20

71. Which one of the following conditions can be treated by means of a sympathectomy?

    (a) Raynaud's disease
    (b) oesophageal varices
    (c) gas gangrene
    (d) varicose ulcer

Chapter 21

72. A cystoscope is

    (a) an instrument used in open surgery on the bladder
    (b) a light carrier used for examination
    (c) a magnifying lens for examination of the ureters
    (d) an instrument used for visual examination of the bladder

73. Obstruction of the urinary tract or failure of urinary peristalsis may result in the condition known as

    (a) pyelonephrosis
    (b) pyelonephritis
    (c) hydronephrosis
    (d) hypernephroma

74. Which of the following malignant growths is *not* found in the kidney?

    (a) retinoblastoma
    (b) Wilm's tumour
    (c) sarcoma
    (d) carcinoma

75. Suppression of urine in a male patient can be due to

    (a) diabetes insipidus
    (b) renal colic
    (c) renal failure
    (d) enlarged prostate gland

76. Which of the following is *not* a varicose vein?

    (a) varicocele
    (b) haemorrhoids
    (c) oesophageal varices
    (d) hydrocele

77. What is orchidopexy?

    (a) a type of fit
    (b) a disorder of speech
    (c) an operation for undescended testicles
    (d) a brain operation

Appendix

78. Match up the X-ray examinations in List 1 with the radio-opaque substances used in List 2

	List 1		*List 2*
A	myelogram	1	diodone
B	cardiogram	2	Hypaque
C	micturating cystogram	3	Pyelosil
D	cholangiogram	4	iodized oil
		5	Myodil

A	B	C	D

79. In a cholecystogram the contrast medium is given by means of

    (a) tablets dissolved in water
    (b) an injection into the circulatory system
    (c) an injection into the biliary tree through a fine cannula
    (d) injection directly into the gall bladder during surgery

Miscellaneous

80. The porter has arrived to take a patient to theatre and the hypodermic premedication has not been given. What should be done?

    (a) give it immediately by hypodermic injection
    (b) give it immediately by intramuscular injection
    (c) inform the theatre porter
    (d) inform the anaesthetist

81. A patient with a diagnosed deep venous thrombosis suddenly develops dyspnoea, chest pain and shock. He is conscious and frightened. Indicate your priority of action from the following list

    (a) administer prescribed heparin and morphine
    (b) administer oxygen
    (c) reassure patient and place in a comfortable upright position
    (d) administer a prescribed oral anticoagulant

1	2	3	4

82. Which of the following intravenous fluids must be given immediately following a blood transfusion (providing intravenous fluids are to be continued)?

    (a) 5% glucose
    (b) Hartmann's solution
    (c) sodium lactate
    (d) sodium chloride

83. Match up the instruments used in List 1 with the conditions the patient is suffering from in List 2

List 1		*List 2*
A bronchoscope	1	hiatus hernia
B sigmoidoscope	2	ulcerative colitis
C gastroscope	3	menorrhagia
D duck-billed speculum	4	foreign body in ear
	5	carcinoma of lung

A	B	C	D

84. Match up the preoperative drugs in List 1 with the adult dosage in List 2

List 1		*List 1*
A Omnopon (H.I.) (papaveretum)	1	0·6 mg
B pentobarbitone (oral)	2	5 mg
C scopolamine (H.I.) (hyoscine)	3	15 mg
D morphine (H.I.)	4	20 mg
	5	200 mg

A	B	C	D

85. Indicate from the following list of
    operations/conditions/treatments the situation when a
    gastric lavage would *not* be carried out

    (a) pyloric stenosis (medical treatment)
    (b) bleeding gastric ulcer
    (c) immediately after swallowing barbiturates
    (d) prior to a partial gastrectomy

86. Match up the pH (acid/alkaline levels) in List 1 with the
    body states or normal fluid pH levels in List 2

	List 1		*List 2*
A	pH 6·9	1	normal blood pH
B	pH 7·3	2	average urinary pH
C	pH 7·4	3	acidosis
D	pH 7·5	4	alkalosis
		5	normal pH of hydrochloric acid in the stomach

A	B	C	D

87. You are in charge of a surgical ward and the following situations occur. Use the match panel to indicate the order in which you should deal with them

    (a) a patient faints in the toilet and is lying on her side
    (b) the consultant surgeon wishes to see you in his office
    (c) a patient's tracheostomy tube has obstructed
    (d) a patient's abdominal wound has burst wide open

1	2	3	4

88. Match up the likely conditions in List 1 with the sites of pain in List 2

List 1		List 2
A appendicitis	1	loin
B renal calculi	2	right shoulder tip
C gastric ulceration	3	epigastric
D cholecystitis	4	right iliac fossa
	5	tip of coccyx

A	B	C	D

89. A steam inhalation is used to

    (a) liquefy secretions in the respiratory passages
    (b) dilate the respiratory passages
    (c) reduce carbon dioxide in the respiratory passages
    (d) stimulate free drainage from the lacrimal apparatus

90. A patient is due out of bed for the first time following
    surgery. Which of the following would indicate that he
    should remain in bed until seen by the doctor?

    (a) sounds 'chesty' but no other signs or symptoms
    (b) blood pressure lower than prior to surgery
    (c) intravenous therapy and gastric aspiration in
        progress
    (d) discomfort in the wound but no sign of inflammation

Answers

Answers

Anatomy and Physiology

1. b
2. d
3. c
4. b
5. b
6. b
7. b
8. d
9. c
10. a
11. b
12. d
13. d
14. c
15. b
16. d
17. c
18. c
19. b
20. d
21. a
22. a
23. d
24. b
25. b
26. d
27. b
28. c
29. c
30. a
31. c
32. d
33. a
34. c
35. b
36. a
37. a
38. d
39. c
40. b
41. c
42. d
43. a
44. b
45. d
46. a
47. d
48. b
49. b
50. c
51. a
52. a
53. b
54. c
55. a
56. c
57. c
58. d
59. b
60. d
61. c
62. a
63. c
64. a

65. c	**Medical Nursing**
66. c	
67. c	1. A4
68. b	B1
69. d	C5
70. c	D3
71. a	2. c
72. a	3. b
73. a	4. A2
74. b	B4
75. d	C3
76. b	D1
77. a	5. d
78. c	6. a
79. b	7. A2
80. a	B4
81. a	C3
82. c	D1
83. c	8. b
84. b	9. a
85. d	10. b
86. a	11. b
87. a	12. b
88. a	13. b
89. b	14. c
90. a	15. c
91. d	16. b
92. b	17. d
93. b	18. c
94. b	19. b
95. b	20. A4
96. a	B5
97. c	C2
98. d	D1
99. d	21. c
100. b	22. c

23.	d	53.	a
24.	b	54.	A3
25.	b		B4
26.	d		C2
27.	c		D5
28.	A3	55.	d
	B5	56.	b
	C2	57.	d
	D1	58.	d
29.	d	59.	d
30.	c	60.	b
31.	c	61.	b
32.	a	62.	a
33.	c	63.	c
34.	a	64.	d
35.	b	65.	b
36.	c	66.	c
37.	b	67.	c
38.	c	68.	d
39.	c	69.	b
40.	c	70.	b
41.	c	71.	c
42.	b	72.	b
43.	a	73.	a
44.	a	74.	b
45.	d	75.	d
46.	c	76.	b
47.	c	77.	a
48.	A2	78.	a
	B4	79.	b
	C3	80.	b
	D5		
49.	c		
50.	b		

Paediatric Nursing

51.	b
52.	d

1. c
2. b

3.	d	39.	c
4.	b	40.	d
5.	a	41.	a
6.	a	42.	d
7.	b	43.	c
8.	c	44.	a
9.	d	45.	a
10.	d	46.	a
11.	c	47.	b
12.	b	48.	c
13.	a	49.	b
14.	c	50.	b
15.	d	51.	c
16.	b	52.	b
17.	a	53.	a
18.	a	54.	b
19.	c	55.	d
20.	c	56.	c
21.	b	57.	b
22.	b	58.	a
23.	c	59.	d
24.	d	60.	a
25.	c	61.	d
26.	b	62.	c
27.	c	63.	a
28.	c	64.	d
29.	a	65.	d
30.	d	66.	b
31.	b	67.	c
32.	d	68.	a
33.	c	69.	b
34.	c	70.	d
35.	a	71.	c
36.	b	72.	b
37.	a	73.	b
38.	c	74.	a

75. d	24. c
76. c	25. a
77. d	26. b
78. b	27. a
79. d	28. c
80. b	29. a
	30. b
Surgical Nursing	31. 1a
1. b	2c
2. A2	3b
B3	4d
C1	32. c
3. b	33. d
4. a	34. a
5. b	35. b
6. a	36. a
7. b	37. b
8. A2	38. c
B3	39. d
C4	40. c
D1	41. c
9. b	42. b
10. c	43. b
11. d	44. A2
12. d	B5
13. c	C1
14. b	D3
15. c	45. a
16. b	46. d
17. c	47. b
18. a	48. c
19. a	49. d
20. d	50. d
21. c	51. b
22. a	52. c
23. a	53. d

54. a
55. b
56. c
57. A3
    B4
    C2
    D1
58. c
59. c
60. a
61. A4
    B2
    C5
    D1
62. d
63. b
64. b
65. b
66. A2
    B4
    C3
    D1
67. b
68. c
69. c
70. b
71. a
72. d
73. c
74. a
75. c
76. d
77. c
78. A5
    B1
    C2

    D3
79. a
80. d
81. 1c
    2b
    3a
    4d
82. d
83. A5
    B2
    C1
    D3
84. A4
    B5
    C1
    D3
    (Any dose less than 1 mg
    must be prescribed in
    micrograms – μg
    1 mg = 1000 μg. There-
    fore a dose of 0·6 mg
    should be prescribed
    600 μg)
85. b
86. A2
    B3
    C1
    D4
    (Explanation of pH scale:

Strongest acid	pH 1
Neutral	pH 7
Strongest alkali	pH 14
Urine	pH 5–8
Blood	pH 7·4
acidosis	pH 7·3
alkalosis	pH 7·5

Hydrochloric acid ranges
pH 1–17)

87. 1c
2d
3a
4b

88. A4
B1
C3
D2

89. a

90. b